Get Hard Again

From Erectile Dysfunction

To Huge Erection

By

Riley Greene

Get Hard Again: From Erectile Dysfunction To Huge Erection

Copyright © 2017

ISBN: 9781520995564

Warning and Disclaimer

Publisher Contact

Skinny Bottle Publishing

books@skinnybottle.com

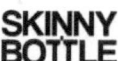

My ED Story

You probably know the feeling, or you wouldn't be reading this right now. That feeling where you are up to bat so to speak and suddenly everything falls short. It's certainly no laughing matter and can definitely leave you feeling a mixture of emotions ranging from anger to depression when erectile dysfunction (ED) becomes all too real for you. For some men, it is merely something that happens once in awhile and really isn't that much of a problem. It's natural not to be able to perform all the time regardless of your age and health. But when the problem of ED becomes an everyday occurrence you can just about make a safe bet that there is something bigger going on.

Because it's just not something that most guys talk about with anybody, let alone one another, I'm going to share with you my personal story of how I was able to overcome my own problems with ED and get myself back to being able to have the same huge erections that I was used to having when I was younger. Don't worry I don't need to go into crazy detail, but I do want you to realize that you aren't alone and that there are a large amount of variations and reasons as to what causes ED. Thankfully, there are just as many ways to respond to ED to get yourself back up and in the game.

Let's start with my story and then we will cover some of the other reasons some men experience ED. For me, it started when I was in my mid-thirties. I must have been around 35 years old. I started to realize that it took me a considerable amount of extra time to get and stay hard. At first, it was something that I could work my way around. The way I viewed it, it gave me more time to spend with my girlfriend, which she didn't seem to really mind. In fact, during those first early years, I was able to do a fairly good job at hiding the fact that I was having a hard time getting it up. It surely wasn't because I wasn't interested in her. It was just that my body didn't seem to want to work like it used to.

Eventually, during our lovemaking, I would be able to complete the job but it still lacked the same level of performance that I had been used to with previous girlfriends. There just was some sort of spark missing. I put off going to the doctor. I knew from reading all sorts of online journals and blogs that I really should commit myself to seeking medical help, but something about going to the doctor made it too real for me. It was like admitting defeat if I were going to walk into the doctor's office and announce that yes, indeed, I was suffering from ED. The breaking point for me was when I realized that I had begun ignoring my girlfriend's sexual needs simply because I didn't want to face the defeat and shame that came along with not being able to perform properly. Eventually, I caved in and made the dreaded doctor's appointment for myself. When I went to the doctor, he ran through what seemed like a standard series of questions for any physical. He asked if I smoked, how much I drank, he wanted to know if I exercised. He also informed me of the extra weight I had put on since I had last been in to see him.

Considering that it had been a couple years I wasn't surprised to see my weight had gone up. It was a bit of a shock that it was thirty pounds up. Then he continued on to ask me if I felt depressed and wanted to know if I was on any anti-depressants or other medications that he was unaware of. He asked me how much I slept and what sort of foods I was eating. I'll be the first to admit that I wasn't eating the healthiest back then. After work and time with the girlfriend I found myself eating mostly manufactured meals that were quick and easy to cook in the microwave. Because they were so small I would usually eat a couple for dinner. Breakfast and lunch were usually covered by some fast food restaurant on my way into work and on my lunch break.

Needless to say, I certainly wasn't eating healthy, though I didn't think that it was the thing that was holding me back in the bedroom. The doctor said there were some tests that he could run on me to rule out whether or not I had developed some sort of circulation problem, but he felt that my main problem was that I had put on weight, had become increasingly less physically active, and wasn't eating properly. Before he did these tests on me he suggested that I simply spend some time putting a little more effort into taking better care of my physical health.

Not quite the reaction I was looking for. Couldn't he just prescribe me some quick pill? There is certainly enough out there on the market. Then he informed me that most insurances don't even cover ED medications without running through a battery of tests to confirm the necessity of medication. In the end, it turned out that the best solution for me was simply to follow the doctor's orders and change my lifestyle. It surely couldn't hurt. It took awhile, maybe about three months before I started noticing any real change in the bedroom department. But, it was certainly starting to go better. Not only did I have more energy in general, but I was also starting to be in better physical shape.

They say that as many as one in four men will experience ED at some point in their life. Scientists are also quick to note that this statistic is also only based on the men willing to have a candid conversation about their performance. Not all men are that quick to admit ED. I know I put off talking to my doctor about it for quite some time. In the end, I'm glad I did and have learned a lot about ED along the way and how you can make your erection harder, bigger, and last longer than ever before. I've tried a lot of products, techniques, and obviously, lifestyle changes and have found the best approach for me has been a combination of all of these. It started with simple lifestyle changes but then I grew into really taking matters of my health seriously. I'm here to pass along some of my knowledge to you so that you can help get back to where you want to be. It is possible, and remember that even though you certainly aren't alone in experiencing ED, it is more than likely something that you can help correct all on your own. Stay strong and determined and you'll get there. I did.

Key Points to Look Forward To

• Non-medical techniques to help you maintain a healthier lifestyle that is designed to help promote increased blood flow and a healthier heart.

• Guidance on which supplements can help the most.

• Tips on how to identify what is causing your own ED.

• The importance of adequate Mental/Emotional Health.

• Tips and Tools that you can use to begin seeing results without a doctor.

• Therapies that are designed to help you open communication with your partner and begin to experience the trust necessary to overcome the defeat that typically accompanies those suffering from ED.

• More advanced medical techniques that are used when you have exhausted all other means.

Garbage Out Healthy Life In

First the Foods

So you probably aware by now that eating right and proper exercise are essential to getting yourself in shape for the bedroom, but what you might not realize is that the types of foods that you eat can have a big impact on your body's circulation. You can actually eat foods that are geared to help you improve blood flow which will help make sure that you are getting harder erections that are more fuller and last longer.

First off think of your dark leafy greens. Kale should quickly become one of your new best friends in the kitchen. You can eat it in a variety of ways including cooking it into soups and one of the more popular ways of making kale chips. Kale chips are simple. You just tear the kale up into bite size pieces (removing the leaf from the stem) and then sprinkle with olive oil and your favorite seasonings and bake at 350 degrees until they are crispy like potato chips. They melt in your mouth and are extremely healthy for you. Plus kale is a relatively inexpensive produce item to stock up on every time you are at the market. Certainly cheaper than buying a bag of potato chips.

Other greens that are good for your heart and blood circulation include broccoli, spinach, and even avocado. The basic rule of thumb is that if it's green you are good to go. Just remember to branch out and try new things other than simply relying on your same old iceberg lettuce.

When you are eating your veggies try to steam them if possible, or eat them raw. Your body gets the highest amount of nutrients from most foods when they aren't overcooked. You may have heard of people that follow a raw diet, and this reason is one of the primary motivators for those willing to make the switch to raw foods. You don't have to go so far as to follow a strictly raw diet or any diet for that matter.

But what you should think about instead, is simply adding more nutritionally sound and healthy choices to your diet. The more you continue to make healthier choices, the quicker you will realize that you don't crave the same old foods. When I first began my healthy eating journey I couldn't imagine going without my doughnuts in the morning with my coffee. Now I have green herbal tea and a bowl of fresh fruit with yogurt. I didn't get there overnight, but eventually, I just stopped craving all the sugary foods.

Along with dark greens, foods such as beets, walnuts, and nuts in general, are all a good source of heart-healthy energy that will make sure your blood is flowing to the right location.

You may be familiar with how nature's shape of foods almost mimics what the food is good for. Like with beets, there rich dark red color is just like the blood flowing through your veins. Eat more of these sweet root vegetables to make sure everything is flowing well.

Beyond choosing your food for its simple ability to specifically help your blood flow, you should also consider cutting out as many processed foods as you possibly can. The simple fact remains that all of the additives, preservatives and other chemicals added to these foods just isn't good for anybody. The food industry makes it difficult sometimes to make the switch to eating more organic simply because the processed foods are less expensive and ultimately more convenient.

I thought I was eating healthy when I was eating my frozen dinners, then I started reading the ingredient lists. My new rule that I follow to a tee is that if I can't pronounce or know what it is, then I just don't eat it. It's pretty simple really but can take some time to make that transition. Don't think that you have to storm through your cupboards and kitchen to clean out everything that may be deemed as 'bad' just realize that next time you go to the market try to pick up some things that are actually good for you.

Once I transitioned over to eating healthier and cooking my own foods or eating them raw I realized that I actually eat less and it's nowhere near as expensive as I once imagined it. Plus I found that you can purchase nice little plastic containers that are inexpensive and great for freezing foods. Now I still have the convenience of having a quick and ready-made meal without the health cost of eating processed foods. My monthly food costs have certainly dropped.

Up and Moving

The other key component to a more healthy lifestyle certainly has to do with the amount of physical activity you get. I found that I personally like setting goals. I needed something that could help me actually monitor and track my movement so I could gauge my daily activity. I'm not here to promote any one device over another, but for me, a wristband that I could link up to my smartphone was the perfect answer. Over the years I've continued to upgrade it and don't ever leave without wearing it. It was nice to know how many steps I took in a day.

At first, my idea of exercising couldn't have been further from what I do now. I essentially did nothing physical. How could I expect to sit around all day on my computer and at work, and then be able to actually perform any sort of physical prowess in the sack? Now it all seems clear, but at the time I just saw my life as this happy routine that had unfortunately fallen way out of the guidelines for an active and healthy lifestyle. Now I actually go to a gym, have a trainer, and have even branched out to doing new things like Yoga.

The main thing exercise does for your body is pretty obvious: it gets you in shape. It helps keep your heart healthy, promotes better blood circulation, and improves your muscle strength and tone. Plus, it boosts your endorphins (those happy feel good chemicals) and helps actually give you more energy. Your exercise levels are something to certainly consider if you are experiencing ED. If for some reason you consider yourself a fit and healthy person that is physically active and still experiencing ED then it is certainly time to make that doctor's appointment to see if there is something else more serious going on with your circulation.

Given the statistics though on how well most of us do on physical activity, the basic assumption is that we all need to exercise more. We live in a time when most of our work is done from a sitting position, along with most of our entertainment (TV. and video games, not to mention time spent on the smartphone perusing our social media). It's just a simple fact that most of us are doing far and far less physically though we are still mentally active and engaged in new ways. The trade off is that our bodies are being neglected. I'm happy to say that I have a girlfriend that loves to get active. She's always down for going for a bike ride or out to play tennis. We even go to the gym together when our schedules match up.

While you can do it all on your own, joining some sort of community of like-minded individuals helps most people get and stay motivated. It's not like you have to tell somebody that you're working out because you have ED. You simply are getting more in shape and staying active. No more reason is necessary. My personal trainer helps make sure that I am always pushing myself and I have found him to be one of the most critical elements I've added to my life. It only costs a few extra dollars for me more a month at my gym and the payoff has certainly been worth it.

In those first few months, I dropped over 50 pounds and am continuing to become more fit and trim daily. Exercise really has boosted my self-confidence, raised my game and made me a lot more assertive in the bedroom. Exercise is a natural testosterone booster and it won't take you long to feel the same sense of power once you start pushing yourself too. Just stay motivated. Do it for yourself. Do it for your partner. Do it for whatever reason. Just get yourself out there and get to it. What's stopping you?

Dietary Supplements

At first, I didn't take any supplements. I felt between eating right and exercising that I was giving my body all that it needed. Then I started reading more and more and talking to more people at the gym about ways to improve my workout performance. I really didn't think that it would also lead to helping me out in the bedroom but I have found that it does.

And the reason why is quite simple. Most of the sport's supplements that are out there are geared to help improve blood flow. They want to make sure that as much nutrient rich blood is engorging your muscles so that you have plenty of fuel to grow bigger and grow longer. The same applies to other regions of the body.

I know there are a lot of sites out there that claim that supplements are all just amped up placebos for people that want something to believe in, but I was doing my best to tackle this beast all on my own and found that I still could use a little boost in the bedroom. I began researching what was in some of the top products on the market and I found that I could essentially by the ingredients on their own for a lot cheaper than buying the product that was made with all the labels promising me a bigger and harder erection. I've also learned that for me, I had to base what worked on actual results.

Many of the reports that I read on supplements would vary so greatly depending on who performed the report that it was ridiculously clear to me that the pharmaceutical companies that produced research on herbal supplements almost always had their hands in results that proved the supplement little better than a placebo. I also found that the websites dedicated to herbal supplements were quite ready to vindictively discredit 'big-farm' and were eager to fight the fight against all pharmaceuticals. There had to be a happy medium.

I personally take a Nitric Oxide booster which helps improve blood circulation, along with a yohimbine supplement, plus a lean whey protein blend for fuel and then I found the two number one things that I could recommend from personal experience: one is a Tribulus Terrestris supplement and the other is red ginseng. The Tribulus supplement is great at releasing bound up testosterone. It's common for men as they age to release less and less testosterone into the blood stream the interesting thing about this is that you are still producing the testosterone it just doesn't go anywhere the older you get. Tribulus is a natural supplement that helps your body release that stored up testosterone in a non-steroidal way. This definitely put me back in the game in many different places in my life.

The red ginseng I have found to be the best at boosting my energy levels and really giving me the stamina in the bedroom that I was looking for. Combined with my daily dose of yohimbine I was getting truly amped up in the area of sexual desire and my erection problems were a thing of the past. Yohimbine I take as a sublingual liquid that I just hold under my tongue. It comes from a tree bark from an African tree and acts similarly to ginseng but I notice a remarkable difference when I forget to take any of my supplements.

Again, I started taking all of these supplements to help my workout and then found that I was suddenly really achieving the rock hard results I was wanting that ED was leaving me without. If you have any sort of blood pressure or heart condition it's always important to check with your doctor. I called my doctor's office and got to speak to my doctor over the phone. He didn't seem to have a problem with any of these supplements for me and advised me just to be smart about following the proper dosage and just monitoring how I felt when I took them. I started all of them on the smallest dose possible and have only increased them slightly over the past year. If it works it works is how I see it, and these supplements work for me. You may want to give them a trial run.

Key Take Away Points

• You are what you eat. If you want to have a healthier sex life you have to have a more robust healthier life all around.

• Learning which foods, such as dark greens and beats, that will help improve your circulatory system and boost your heart health.

• Learning to avoid processed foods.

• Following a smart plan of exercise.

• Learning that you don't run a marathon overnight. You have to build your physical health up from whatever starting point you are at.

• Determining if supplements are right for you.

• Learning that when it comes to treatment for ED you have to discover what works for yourself above and beyond what any of the critics say.

You are What You Think

Just like maintaining a healthy lifestyle can help boost your sex drive the same can be said about the things that you are thinking about. As my downward spiral to full-blown ED began I found myself continually stressed out every time that it was my turn to do the deed. It was like I knew that I was going to fail and couldn't even get the pleasure of being able to actually enjoy myself. So how does one stop the perpetual anxiety that starts to kick in once you feel alienated from your member? Well for starters you have to train your self-talk. It's almost like pulling a con on yourself. You have to build yourself up a bit and focus more on pleasuring your partner and actually enjoying yourself. Sex is like life, it's more about the journey than the destination. If you kick back and allow yourself the patience to perform at your own speed you will be surprised how much this can make a difference.

The next thing to do is remember that your partner is with you. If you are worried about not being big enough or hard enough then you certainly won't be able to actually perform any good. Give yourself the enjoyment that comes with knowing that your partner has accepted you for who you are and that you are already good enough.

If these things continue to fail you there are some other things you can do to mentally get your nether regions swirling with rock hard blood flow. For starters, if you masturbate a lot then masturbate less. If you don't masturbate at all start doing it. The point is, is that you need to shake things up for your body. If you are constantly jerking off than odds are you probably just don't have the stamina to dedicate yourself to your partner on top of all the self-pleasure you've been indulging in. Plus, if you still have plenty of seed to spill, then just work on changing up the ways that you masturbate. Invest in a Fleshlight or something similar that gets you in the habit of using your pelvic thrusts to get you off as opposed to just merely relying on your hand. You would be surprised what a big difference it makes when you practice hands-free masturbation. It certainly gets you in the mood for the real thing, plus makes a pretty good workout.

If you are more the type that doesn't masturbate at all then you really can't expect your penis to know what's going on when it comes time to actually use it. You could simply be overly sensitive when it comes time to perform. While you might think that will make you better and harder it can actually have the adverse effect. What constitutes masturbating too much or too little, well only you can know. On average most grown men masturbate once every day or two. That means a few times a week. Of course, for others, they may go at it two or three times a day and still be able to perform adequately. You have to gauge for yourself what exactly is too little or too often. Just remember to not neglect your own needs while at the same time not overly indulging. Save some of that juice for your main squeeze.

Giving into Your Fantasies

Another thing I have noticed that has made a big difference in my capacity for a raging boner is how far I let myself go into my fantasies. There were so many times in my past where I would simply be giving my girlfriends what I thought they wanted. It was enough to get the job done (until it wasn't) but I still wasn't actually doing the things that I imagined doing. For me I like a little bondage and some light BDSM, that may seem like too much information, but stick with me I do have a point here. The reason I share this is because so often I treated my girlfriends like they were some sort of fragile pristine glass that would shatter under my

14

full force. I was essentially always holding myself back. What's worse is that they would tell me to let go and relax, but I still couldn't bring myself to fully express myself sexually. Now with the added confidence, I have built I am able to be more forceful in the bedroom, nothing any more than your standard Fifty Shades of Grey, but still enough to allow me to take control and play the dominant role that I personally prefer to wear. I have found that the sex that I have is far better these days and is a far cry from the sex I've had over the past few years when I was meek and mild in my lovemaking.

Who knows what your fantasies are. Only you do. But you should definitely allow yourself the capacity to actually follow through with some of them and see just how well your partner is into the same thing. It's always a good idea to have a light conversation about what you both imagine doing to each other before you just dive in with the whips and bondage straps. But the conversation can be light and playful and full of the reminder that the whole point of sex is to enjoy one another on a fully open level. If you aren't able to do that with your partner, you just might be with the wrong person. But you never know until you open up and express yourself. Give it a try.

To Porn or Not to Porn

While it's very true that just about every guy likes watching porn, you might not realize the negative effects that it can have on your ability to get and maintain an erection when you are actually in the driver seat. For starters, there is nothing wrong with watching porn in and of itself. It only becomes a problem when it becomes a problem, for many a man this is when they are unable to actually achieve an orgasm without having the extra visual stimulation of porn.

You should be able to have just a good orgasm without the need of porn as you do when you enjoy it. While some couples are able to bring porn into their sexual life as a couple, you don't want to have to rely on pressing play on a video every time you need to get it up. A good practice if you find yourself caught up in the sticky goo of watching too much porn is to simply work on rubbing one out with no porn.

Close your eyes and think about how good it feels to touch yourself and imagine that your partner is the one that is touching you. Let the porn that plays in your mind's eye be the sort of porn that you are able to recreate in your own life. This sort of practice helps get and keep you in the moment of being connected to your body. It's easy when watching a porn to put yourself in the shoes of the dude banging away, but you aren't connecting with your own body. If anything you are distancing yourself by placing yourself in a fantasy that is just not realistic or even possible.

For starters, you aren't him. Which brings us to the next negative effect that porn plays on your mental gymnastics. It's easy to start to compare yourself to others in porn. Maybe if you are like the average man with a 5-inch penis, you realize quickly that you just don't measure up to the men in most porn. There's a reason why they are in the porn industry and believe it or not, a lot to do with how big and hard they are has to do with drugs, camera angles, and lots of takes to get just that perfect shot. It's a business that is in the business of selling sex.

Of course, it's over-indulgent. It's there to fulfill fantasies, not showcase the ugly reality of a guy trying to shove a limp hose in a dry hole. Take yourself out of the porn fantasy and focus more on making your own relationship better. For starter's if it's a dry hole, go down on her for awhile. Get things flowing first before you try jumping right in. You probably know this already, but just in case you didn't there's a quick tip for you.

Don't think I'm trying to come down hard on avid porn fans. It's just a simple fact that too much outside visual stimulation can flood your mind with images of sex acts that you either down live up to, or would rather be having than the one that is coming up short. If you just give yourself a break from it from time to time, you will be surprised at the swift balance back that your member makes in responding to your touch and to that of your partners.

Key Take Away Points

- Watch your self-talk.

- Take time to focus on your own pleasure.

- Follow through with your fantasies.

- Be mindful when you take time to watch porn.

- Be careful not to over indulge.

Some Actual Exercises

Aside from actually working out at the gym, there are some actual exercises that you can do that specifically focus on your penis and can help make you harder, bigger, and last a lot longer when it comes to getting huge. The number one exercise that you will see and hear from doctors and sex experts is doing kegel exercises. In case you don't know what these penis workout exercises are it's where you tighten your pelvic floor just like you do when you are urinating and have to stop the flow midstream.

Clenching and releasing this muscle continually throughout the day helps strengthen the muscles that are responsible for helping you maintain a firm erection. Along with continually 'pulsing' this muscle, it's important to tighten and hold it for as long and hard as you can before releasing. The best thing about this exercise is that you can do it anytime of the day, anywhere that you are, and nobody has to even know that you are secretly working out your penis. Just don't forget to do them frequently and often. At least three sets a day.

The Jelq

The jelq, or rather jelqing, is an amazing workout that can take some real dedication of time and energy to complete and isn't for the weak of determination. You have to be strong, be able to hold back your orgasms, and dedicate a significant amount of time (about an hour) to each jelqing session. It is an old technique that has been around and secretly coveted for many years but has begun to surface and gain more exposure as people realize how much potential this exercise has for making results, results that are measurably different.

The just of jelqing is that you are going to engorge the blood vessels in the shaft and head of your penis and continually work on maintaining them so that they can grow in size and take on more blood. More blood means harder erections that are also bigger. Win-win if ever there was one. And you don't really need any tools. Just some coconut oil or cocoa butter and a hot washrag (and a lot of stamina).

The first step is to warm your penis up. Just the same way that you wear a hot towel on your face to open your pores before you shave, the same applies to the theory behind warming your penis up. You are preparing the blood vessels to accept more blood. The easiest way to do this is with a wash rag. Sit on the edge of your tub (or grab a chair if you only have a shower unit) and warm your towel up as hot as you can stand it. Remember you aren't trying to burn yourself, but you should be able to manage a significant amount of heat. Ring the water out of your washrag and drape or wrap it around your cock. Sit there with it until it starts to get cool and then do this again. You should do this for anywhere between 5 and 10 minutes before you are ready to actually begin jelqing.

The next step to your jelqing session, just like any exercise, is to do some light stretching to get your penis ready for the serious workout you are just about to give it. To do the stretches you want to grab penis with a dry towel, your dry hand, or even a t-shirt. Grab it just about an inch or so back from the head. You want to remember that the head is sensitive and you don't want to ruin any sensitivity to the head.

Once you have a firm grip on your penis pull it straight out from your body. You should feel a little tightness but you don't want to pull to the point that you are in pain. Pain will only cause you setbacks in your growth and hardness. Just like beginning exercises of any kind you have to start somewhere and work your way up. Hold your penis in an outward position for about 30 seconds. Then you will proceed to pull it out to the left, then to the right, straight up, and straight down. You will want to at least 3 sets of these every time before and after you do you jelqing.

The actual jelqing process is quite simple but highly effective. You begin by grabbing your penis at the base with your ring and thumb forming a tight grip around it. Your grip should be tight enough to push the blood flow down as you begin your stroke, but again not too tight that you are in pain. Then proceed to move your grip down to the end of your shaft right before you reach the head. As you reach the head you will want to grab your penis with your other hand and begin another jelq. As you work your shaft keep switching from hand to hand so that you can keep the blood flow pumping into your penis where it can engorge those warmed up blood vessels.

When you do your jelqs each one should last just a couple seconds and you should always use some sort of lubrication. Many people like cocoa butter or coconut oil because of the unique way that these two natural lubes help heal and maintain healthy skin quality. They also last a long time which will carry you through the standard jelqing session which should last you anywhere from 5 minutes in the beginning on up to 10-15 minutes as you begin to get more experienced.

It's really important that you don't cum when you are doing your session. You will probably get yourself close several times during your first few sessions. In fact, if you find yourself getting more than half-hard then you need to take a quick breather until your erection goes down. You don't want to jelq a fully hard dick. It's counter effective to causing the stretching and hardness improvement that you are aiming for.

When you have completed your jelqing session you proceed to begin your cool down session which is just like any other workout. You need to do another 3 sets of stretching followed by another warm washrag session where you rest your worked out member. Eventually, you will get more comfortable with the feel of jelqing and will find that you can push yourself harder and longer, just remember you don't get there overnight. It takes time, dedication and stamina.

A Tool for Your Tool

Some exercises require a little added assistance. If jelqing seems like a little too much work for you, you can always turn to the classic penis pump. The penis pump or penis vacuum has been used by men for quite a long time to help them achieve erections that are larger and harder. Some argue that it can decrease your sensitivity but if you use it correctly by not overdoing it the device itself is fairly harmless.

The way it works is quite simple. The device is a plastic tube that has a base cock ring on it, a tube at the top that runs to a hand pump that you use to pump the air out of the plastic tube once your penis is inside it.

Next, you just simply insert your penis, pump away with the hand pump, and watch as your penis grows to fill the tube. Once you have reached the size and hardness you are going for then you simply let the air out of the tube from a release valve located on the top and the cock ring that sits at the base of the pump now serves to help you keep your penis hard and engorged. It really is quite simple

A lot of guys think that it takes the fun out of being able to randomly have spontaneous sex, but not being able to have sex at all is a lot worse than taking a few quick minutes to pump it up. Plus, many men that use pumps a few times find that they really don't need to use it that often. It is something that helps get the blood flowing once again and can keep it flowing. Plus, they're just plain good old fashioned fun to use. They should be in your assortment of sex toys even if you don't have ED. Just be sure to follow the directions to a tee that come with the device as the number one result of injury from using penis pumps is a direct result of not paying attention to following the directions. Also, just like with jelqing it doesn't hurt to do a few warm up stretches as well as applying a warm towel for a few minutes to make sure all the blood is up and flowing before you pump away.

Key Take Away Points

- Jelqing helps build and maintain your erections.

- Kegels can build the strength of your erections.

- Use a penis pump to help you get going.

What ED is Not

Dispelling the Myths

Because ED is something that men don't really talk about there are several myths surrounding it, most of them built out of companies that rely on men's secrecy to sell their own products at 'curing' ED. One of the number one myths is that there is one specific cure-all that will make you rock hard whenever and wherever you want. Sure you could go the pharmaceutical route, and we will talk about that in a little bit, but often times that route is expensive and just doesn't stand its ground as an option for most men. That leaves lots of room for natural dietary supplements that are designed to give you the boost you need to make you harder and bigger. Many of these products all contain the same products, and while some of them can help you, the truth is that there are so many components that go into why a man is experiencing ED. There is a combination of psychological and physiological elements that when combined often result in ED. Therefore there just isn't one simple fix-it-all that is even possible. Studies have shown that as few as 18 million men experience ED at some point in their life. Plus if you think that just because you have experienced ED once that you are now going to have it frequently you couldn't be further from the truth. Nobody can perform all the time. Most guys just don't talk about it. But if you experience ED for several months at a time than you are probably a candidate to talk to you doctor about what is going on.

Because it's a combination of things, your doctor can help you determine whether you are simply too stressed out, not eating correctly, not exercising enough and your doctor can even do some simple blood tests to rule out low testosterone levels or to see if there is any problem with your blood pressure. There are certainly some hard and true physical reasons why you can't get it up, but for most people that experience ED it is a combination of mentally losing confidence, being stressed or overworked, and then not taking proper care of the body.

Keeping a journal of when you experience ED can greatly help you determine what is going on. Write down what you eat every day and then mark days that you experience ED. Note if you worked extra hours or were stressed about life events. Try to be as detailed as you can as to what was going on each day. This process of keeping a journal can help you when you do decide to finally go the doctor. It's a lot easier for a doctor to take a look at a running ledger of what you have been experiencing than for you to try to recall any substantial long-term information.

Viagra is the Cure

Many men think that all they need is a prescription for Viagra, Cialis, Levitra or any of the other ED medications to get them back up and running. First off as mentioned earlier there isn't one simple cure. That aside, medications such as these are often times the last resort and just aren't handed out without a doctor determining that they are absolutely necessary. They also work differently. Some of them take an hour to take effect while others take up to two hours. It's not like you just pop a pill and then suddenly are ready to perform.

While medication can help your body's muscles relax enough to get the blood flowing, they can't solve the stress in your life, and certainly won't make your lovemaking magically become better. You have to put work into living a healthier more efficient life that is packed with lots of physical activity and healthy foods. You can't expect to just eat fast food every day and then pop a pill whenever you want to get it up. Not that you necessarily feel that way, but some guys do. The ones that think that is the way things work in for a shocking surprise when their doctor tells them to drop weight and quit smoking.

Speaking of smoking, it is extremely bad for your erectile health. So is drinking. Boo, right? Where's the fun in that? You may think that smoking and drinking actually decreases your stress, but the stress that it puts on your body makes it so that your penis is left with little to no access to the blood flow it needs to get it up. It has been found that as many as one-quarter of all smokers experiencing ED that quit smoking regained substantial erections. That's one in four. Definitely, an easy way to boost your penile health without having to pop a pill or pay a doctor. Plus, you save a lot of money when you quit smoking. Money you can spend on a gym membership. Get a trainer.

Not trying to sound harsh, but a lot of men believe that their bad habits don't have any affect on them. As men, we like to believe we are like Superman, that we can get away with anything without having to pay the price. Also, just because you can't get it up once or twice it doesn't mean that you necessarily have ED. ED is not the same as not being able to perform. ED has to occur for a long period of time before you can actually be diagnosed with it. Sure, a few failed performances are likely to lead any man to believe that his days of lovemaking are numbered, but rest assured that with a few lifestyle changes you can more than likely regain what you have been missing out on.

Key Take Away Points

- ED is not just a problem with your penis.

- Keep a journal.

- Medications don't necessarily solve the problem.

- Keep bad habits in check.

Beyond the Doctor

Seeking a Sexual Therapist

Sometimes the problems that cause ED lean far more into the psychological aspects of the guy that's having a hard time performing in the bed. Going to a Sex Therapist can actually be worth it to help you get to the bottom line of what is causing your problems. Here are a few things that you can expect when you go to see a therapist and what you should look for in a good one.

For starters, you should consider yourself a prime candidate for sex therapy if you are still waking up with morning wood, or if you are able to get an erection on your own. This means that at least all your parts are still working, they just aren't working when and where you want them to. A therapist will help expose you to different aspects of sexuality and teach you to communicate your needs better with your partner so that you can get back to doing the thing you really want to do.

When you begin sessions you will most likely find that your therapist provides you with a substantial amount of 'homework' to do. The counselor will more than likely give you books that you can read that will teach you about the importance of being in touch with your sexuality. This may sound like a bunch of hippy tree-hugging mumbo jumbo, but stick with what the counselor is sharing with you and know that it is going to help you get in touch with your own sexuality.

The therapist will also more than likely give you a variety of exercises that involve touching yourself as well as your partner that are created to help you take away the added pressure to take touching right directly into sexual penetration. You are essentially learning how to be sensual and to slow down and enjoy the process of intimacy as opposed to merely jumping right into the finale. For many men, this helps remove the pressure to perform and allows them to experience a much more intense sexual experience.

Even if you are experiencing ED symptoms as a result of something more physical than mental, it is important that you still seek the aid of a therapist. ED can cause a wide array of personal stress and pressure that can affect you personally as well as the state of your relationship. Trained professionals can work with couples to help guide them through the process of going from a relationship that is lacking in physical intimacy. There is a process of opening up to one another again after one partner experiences ED. The results of ED effect both members of the relationship. Trained therapists are specially trained to help you recognize areas that you may have grown apart from each other and will help facilitate the growth back to a healthy relationship.

Sex therapy is generally a short treatment of around 20 appointments or sessions and generally has a high success rate. A good therapist will also be trained to recognize if you are suffering from something more serious like depression or anxiety issues that may require medication and more intensive counseling to help get you back to a state of stability. Now let's take a look at some of the exercises you might just encounter.

The Blindfold

So you might think of a blindfold as something closer to whips and bondage, but really it can be used as a means of enhancing your sensual pleasure for both yourself and your partner. The ultimate goal of a successful lovemaking session is to be able to physically please both of yourselves. When you use a blindfold you eliminate one of the senses that can sometimes get in the way of establishing a powerful sexual style.

Start by deciding who gets to where the blindfold first and agree that you will only initiate sexual intercourse if your partner gives you a signal such as rubbing your genitals. Keep things light and try to enjoy exploring your partner's body without them being able to see you do it. Feel free to use a free hand to stimulate yourself. Explore what it feels like to enjoy the pleasure of watching your partner moan and become pleasured by your touch. If things lead on further than they do, but there shouldn't be any expectation of things to go forward.

Next, try switching it up and you wear the blindfold. Let your partner's touch be the guide for your sexual pleasure while you sit back and enjoy the ride. Let yourself let go of having to be in control and see where things go. You may find that you are standing at full attention and throbbing with anticipation as you wait to feel what your partner does next to you.

Never underestimate the power of the blindfold. You don't have to do this exercise lying down either. In fact, it's best if both partners are in a sitting position so that the one wearing the blindfold is in front, and the other is behind them cradling them. This position takes away the pressure to perform and ensures that the person being blindfolded feels safe and at ease. This can open up channels of passion and intimacy that are often neglected when simply trying to jump right into sexual intercourse.

Keep Your Relationship Clean

Because so much of sexual performance is based on your level of trust and intimacy with your partner you have to ask yourself if you are keeping the relationship clean with one another. If the two of you can't seem to get along well outside of the bedroom then why would you expect yourself to actually be able to just flip a switch and instantly be available at the drop of a dime. The truth is that you need to keep lines of communication open.

This isn't just about keeping your cock raging hard, it's about making sure that you actually feel openly connected and turned on by your partner. If they are doing something that is bothering you the worst thing you can do is think that you can just go to bed and 'sleep on it'. You should try to resolve issues as soon as they become apparent. This way you build an intensely more honest and open relationship that is built on honesty and trust.

You might not think that this would effect you in the bedroom, but if you feel your partner is always nagging you and telling you what to do you might start to lose your sense of power in the bedroom. You need to be able to stand up for yourself and take charge of things. Most women want a man that is capable of doing that in more places than just the bedroom. Don't be afraid to assert yourself.

When it comes time to articulating yourself do your best not to point fingers or place blame. Express something in terms of how it makes you feel and ask your partner why they are behaving in the way that they are. The more you let things boil up inside of you the harder it will be to express them and the further it will drive the two of you apart.

Once you get comfortable with expressing yourself to your partner, you will begin to notice that you will start to be more open the morning after a sexual encounter to discuss things that you both enjoyed the experience and perhaps places where you felt it could have been better. Open communication is a way to help you prevent the pressure that comes from anticipating your partner's needs while also helping you to be able to meet your own needs.

Try to give yourselves at least one hour a day where you are both completely free to express to each other whatever it is that want without having to worry about any repercussions of what is said. This is your time to express your truth while also giving your partner time to express their own truth. The important thing to remember during this honesty hour is that you need to respect your partner and not say things in a hurtful manner. Be courteous but stand your ground as to what it is you have to say.

Key Take Away Points

- Sex therapy can help.

- Focus more on intimacy and less on the actual act of penetration.

- Be sure to keep the relationship free from drama.

Other Medical Options

There are some cases of ED that just don't seem to be resolved through any amount of healthy eating, exercise, and counseling. For these cases, there is usually an underlying medical issue that is causing the problem. It can be a problem with your actual penis or it could be something more easily treatable such as low testosterone levels. A doctor will clearly be able to run the tests to help you know what the problem is when other treatment methods have been exonerated. Just to let you know what sort of treatment you may be looking at here are a few of the more common treatments.

Testosterone Treatments

Hormone treatments are about five percent of all the treatments in most ED cases. That means a very small percent of the large percent of men experiencing ED are actually a result of low testosterone. If however, your levels are low, you can get treatments from your urologist that will range from injections to patches you place directly on your ball sack. Low testosterone levels usually are accompanied by a dramatic decrease in sexual desire. Still, though, blood testing is required to be clear.

This may seem like a quick fix for a serious problem, but it does come with some downsides. For starters, it has been shown to enlarge the prostate. This means that you run the risk of developing prostate cancer and facing frequent urination problems. Nothing says sexy like having to rur to the bathroom every fifteen minutes to pee. It can also make your balls shrink, much the same way that taking steroids can. For some men, the payoff is worth it considering that they are able to regain the sex life that they once had despite having small balls and an engorged prostate.

Give It a Shot

Before we start talking about penile implants there is always the possibility of self-injection therapy. Yep, you heard that right. You inject your own penis with a shot. Sounds horrendous, doesn't it? Well, the truth is it really isn't all that painful. The needles are really fine and you are taught to put them into a place on the penis that really has relatively minimal nerve endings. If anything the medicine may cause a little burning but that doesn't happen with every case.

Erections from self-injections usually last up to an hour and can even last long after you cum which means you can keep going for longer to make sure your partner is fully satisfied. Clearly, self-injections aren't nearly as invasive as having implants, but there are a few downsides aside from the fact that you're giving yourself a shot in the penis.

The main downside is that in some men the area where the shot is inserted can begin to develop scar tissue. The scar tissue effects the way an erect penis looks and is not reversible. There is also a risk of having an erection that just won't go away. Any erection that lasts longer than four hours requires a trip to an emergency room (or your doctor if you are lucky enough to have them available). It may sound like a fun thing to have an erection that long, but it can cause long-term damage to your penile tissue and that is definitely not something you want to live through.

Going Inside

As a last ditch effort, your urologist may decide that you are a candidate for penile implants. Penile implants offer great satisfaction to men that have exhausted all other means of trying to get and maintain and erection. The implants aren't designed to make you any bigger or wider than you already are, but they are designed to help give you on-demand erections without the need for having to worry about having to self-inject or run into the other room to grab your penis pump. This is definitely a perk for the man looking to truly improve his sex life.

It works by inserting to long cylinders down both sides of the penis. Then these are connected to a pump that is inserted into your scrotum. Next, a reservoir is put into an area that is underneath the groin area. The way it works is by pumping the pump in your scrotum, a saline solution then flows from the reservoir to the cylinders. The result: a rock hard erection. When you are finished having sex all you have to do is pump your balls again and the erection will go away. The process most men find quite simple and relatively painless as far as procedures go. Though as with all medical procedures, there are some slight risks and relative downsides to penile implants.

One of the main downsides is that as many as ten percent of all implants break within five years. For many men, this is a risk that they willing to take considering that nothing else has been able to work for them.

There is also the issue of the head of the penis. The implant shafts only run down the sides of the penis that means if you can't get an erection then really only the sides of your penis will be hard. It will still be enough to get you hard enough for penetration, but you may feel that your penis looks a little smaller since the head isn't full of blood. For many men once they get going, blood eventually finds its way into the head, it just might not be right at first like you would wish it to be.

On a plus note, nobody knows that you have penile implants unless you tell them. Nobody will be able to look at you and tell the difference.

You'll be fine in the locker room just as well as the bedroom. For many men, this is a win-win situation after suffering so much defeat with every other kind of treatment.

Key Take Away Points

- Medication may be necessary

- Testosterone therapy may help.

- Self-injections are a possibility.

- Implants are the last resort.

Enjoy!

Knowing your body is the key to being able to figure out what exactly is causing your ED. For many men, the root is something much more psychological than it is physical. While ED can be a symptom of something much more serious, such as heart disease, you shouldn't jump to assumptions thinking that you are going to have a heart attack anytime soon.

Yes, you should seek medical advice to make sure that the root of your problem isn't something physical, but don't be surprised when you come back with a clean bill of health and still don't know what is going on with your member.

Hopefully, you don't have to go through the process of having to self-inject or go so far as to get implants. I have to say for me I was glad to learn that I had more of an issue with the fact that I hadn't been taking proper care of myself. I don't know why it took a doctor to get me to see that I wasn't eating right or exercising, but my body was certainly letting me know. If you take the time to take a serious look at the way you are living and what your lifestyle is like then you might find the answer to your own problems with ED.

Every man is different. Just don't give up hope that you have lost your ability to get hard. It's a myth that as you age you lose your erection. I'm still going strong and now that I am taking better care of myself I am in fact going stronger than ever before. There's no reason that you can't too. You just have to discover the root of your problem and go from there.

Stay strong and remember to enjoy yourself.

Did you know you could leave an anonymous Amazon review?

If you enjoyed this book, and would like to help make cuckolding more understood and accepted, please consider leaving a review on Amazon. If you are concerned about privacy, you can always use a pen name other than your name. You can change your pen name in a few seconds by following these video instructions:

https://www.youtube.com/watch?v=p5IrU3nPivs

Win a free

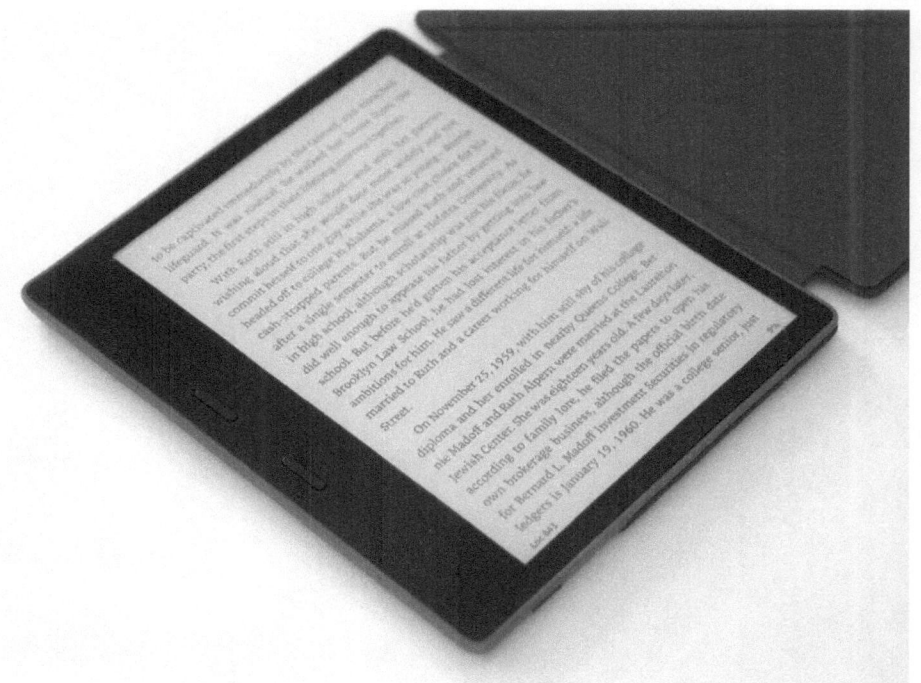

kindle
OASIS

Let us know what you thought of this book to enter the sweepstake at:

http://booksfor.review/hardagain